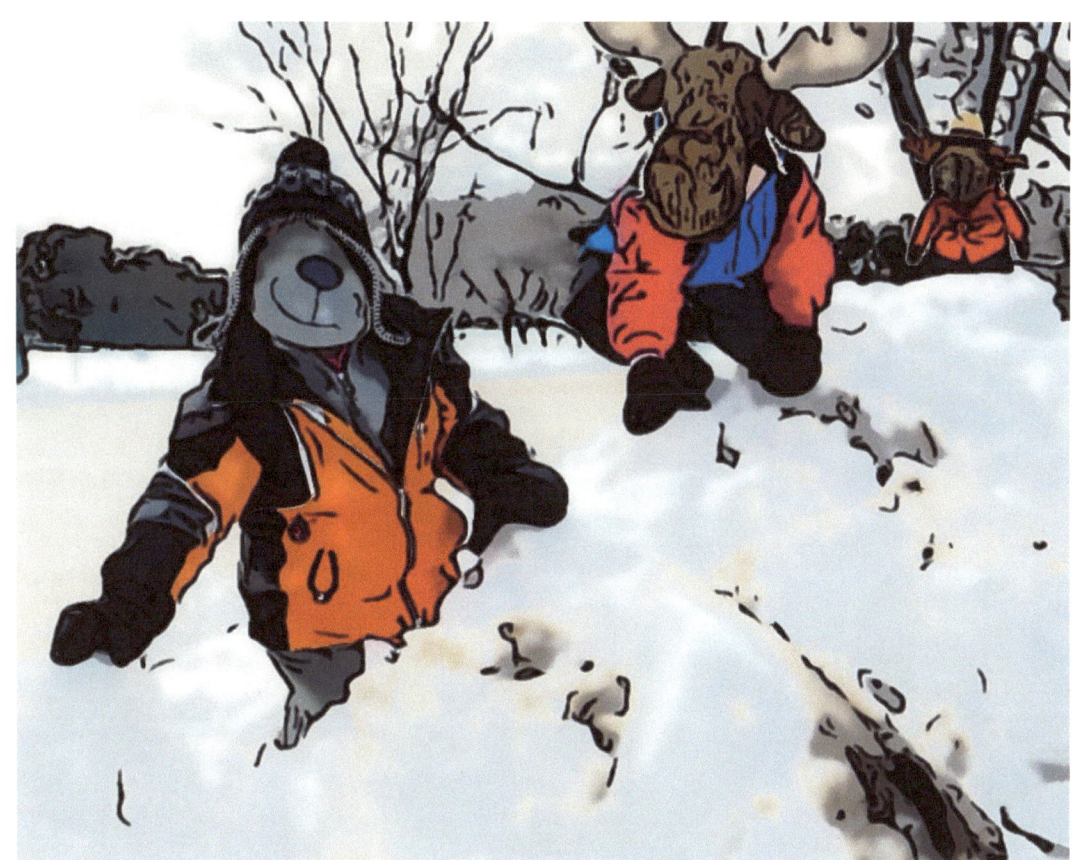

The Moose With The Pump

A book about Type 1 diabetes

By

Yerachmiel Altman & The Moose with the Pump

published by CreateSpace

© 2018 Yerachmiel Altman

All rights reserved. No portion of this book may be reproduced in any form without permission from the author, except as permitted by U.S. copyright law.

For permissions contact: YBA613@hotmail.com

ISBN-13: 978-1540709981

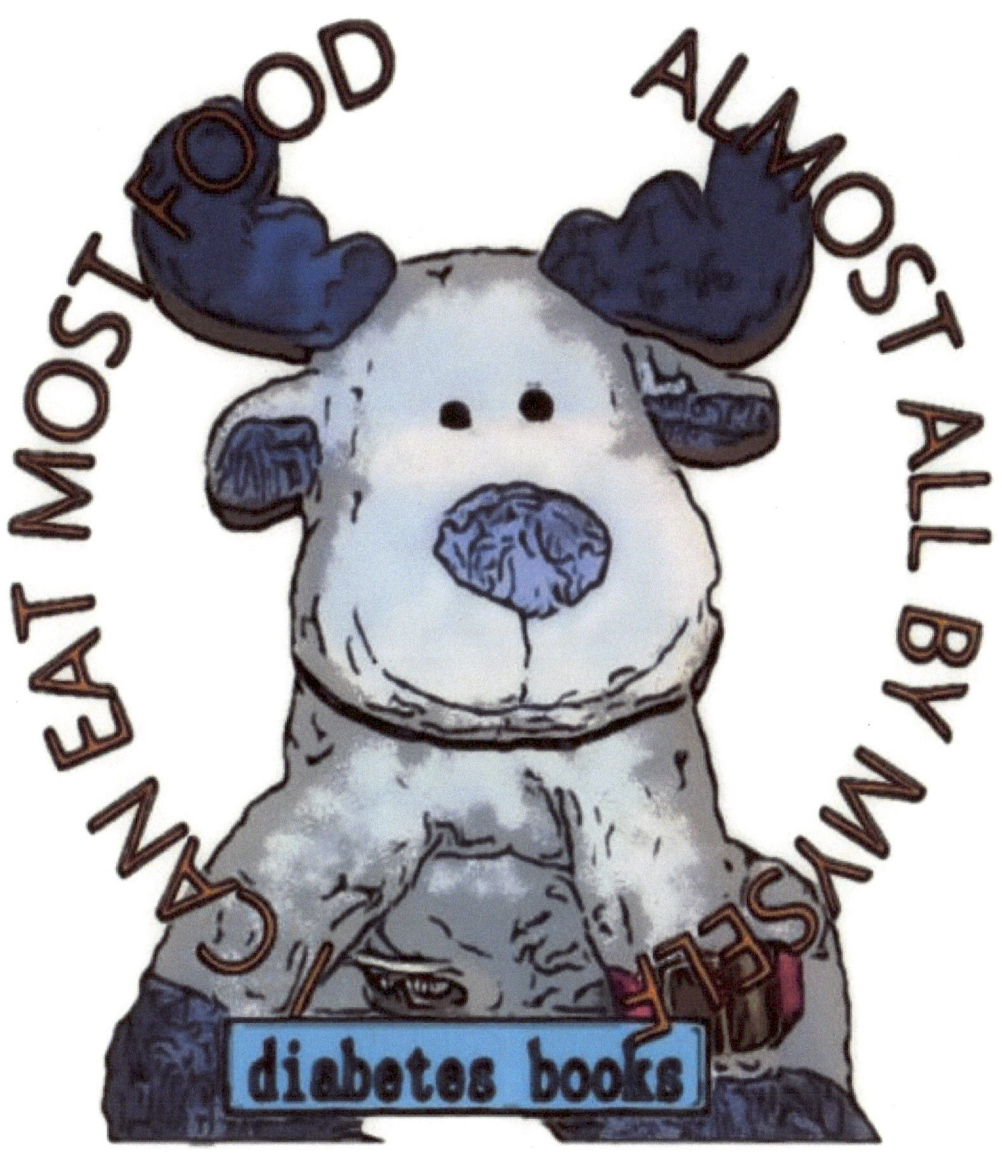

My name is David Jacob,
   A little blue moose am I.
My doctor said I have diabetes,
   And said no one knows why.

My parents learned about it,
   To take blood tests and give a shot.
My new pump helps keep sugar level,
   And my sensor alarms when it's not.

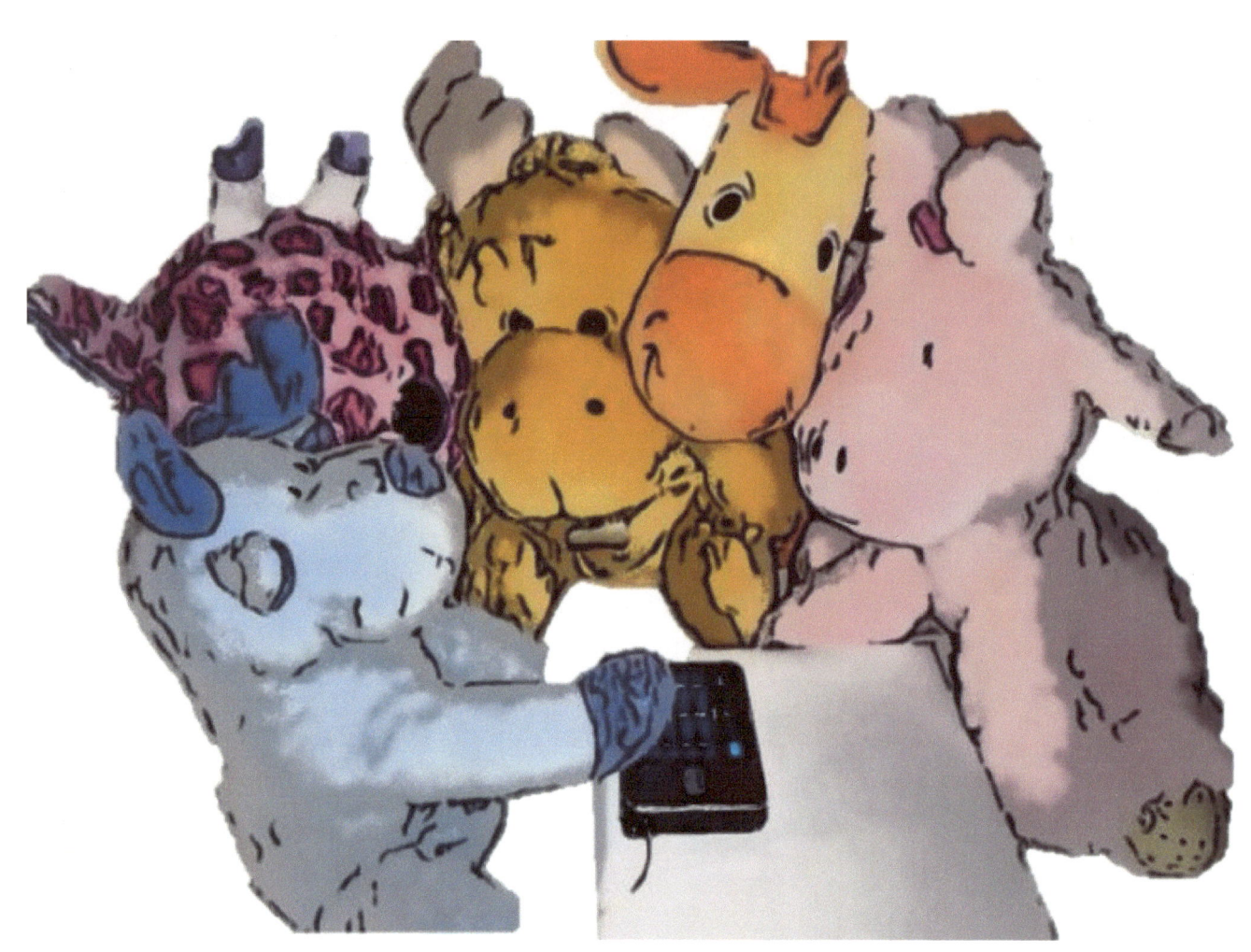

"Have no fear," said my parents,
 "We will not let you down.
With the right information,
 You'll be safe and sound."

"We will not let you fall,
 Or not know what to do.
As we learn new things,
 We will share them with you."

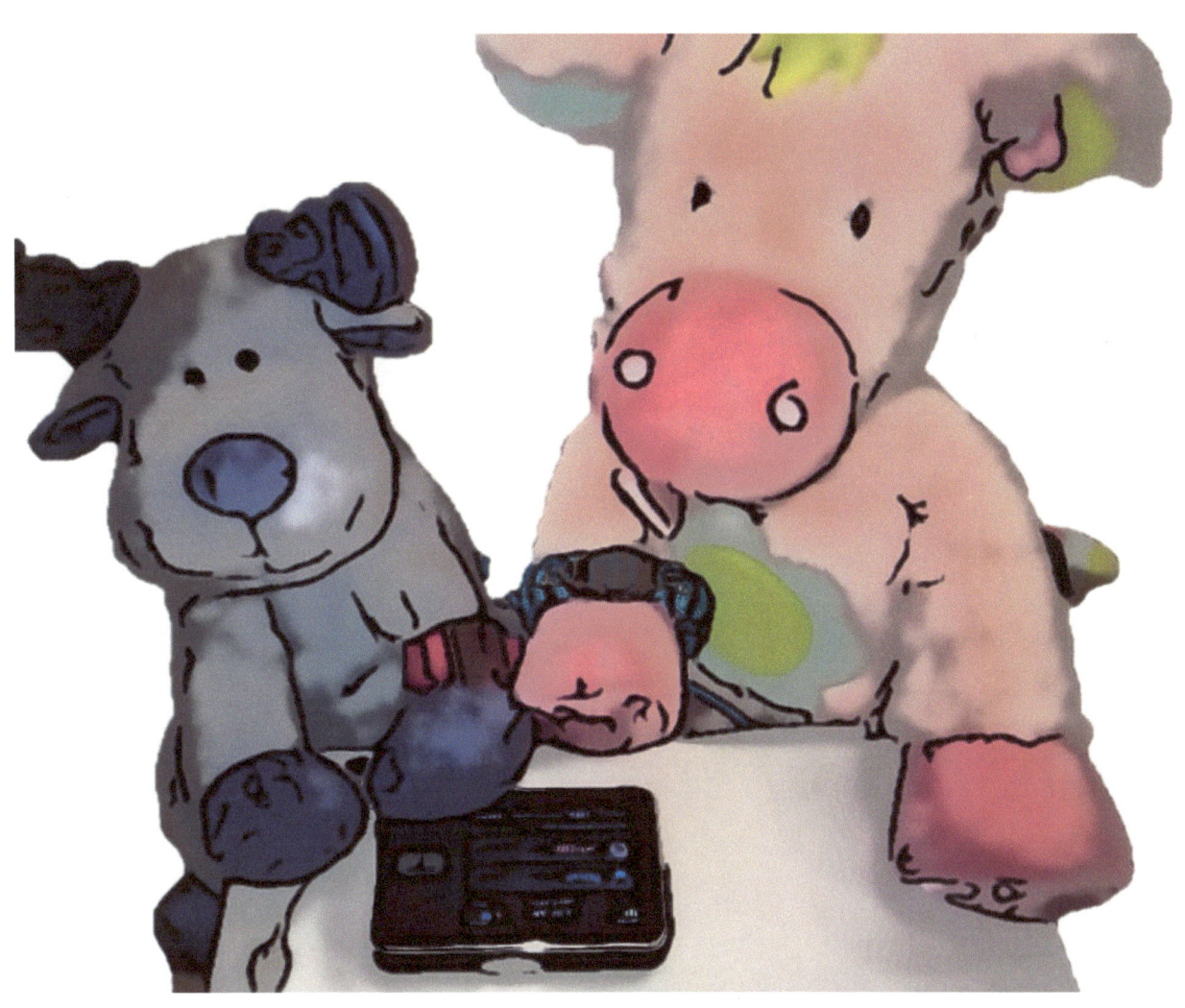

"We will help you to learn
    To keep your sugar good all day,
Using shots, blood tests,
    Pumps and sensors", they did say.

My big sister Adina
    Learned to take care of me too.
And now together we will be
    Sharing everything with you.

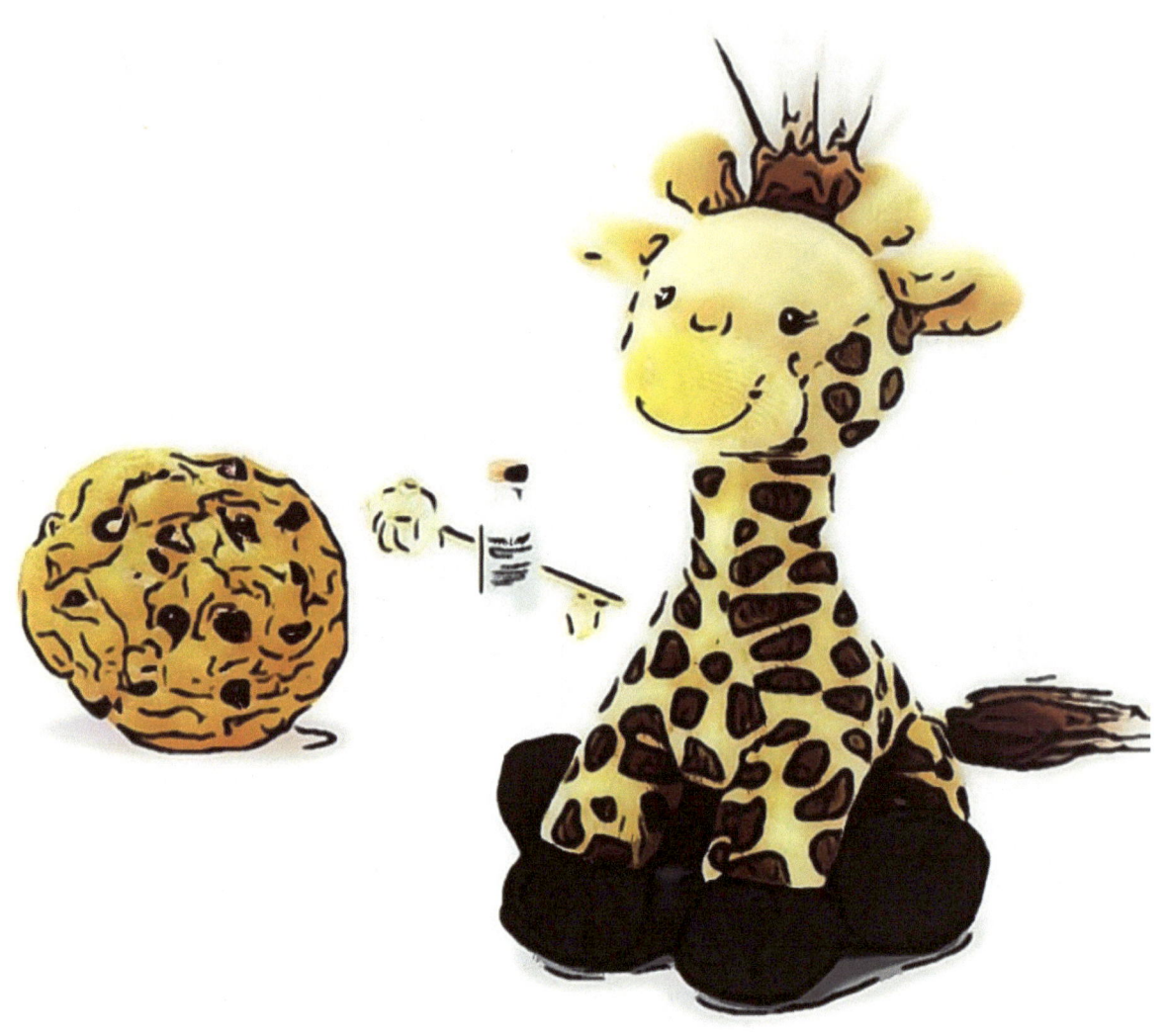

Food needs insulin
   To give us energy to play.
With diabetes have to get
   Insulin another way.

We balance food and actions,
   With insulin we feel well.
If we don't get it right,
   The sensor's alarm will tell.

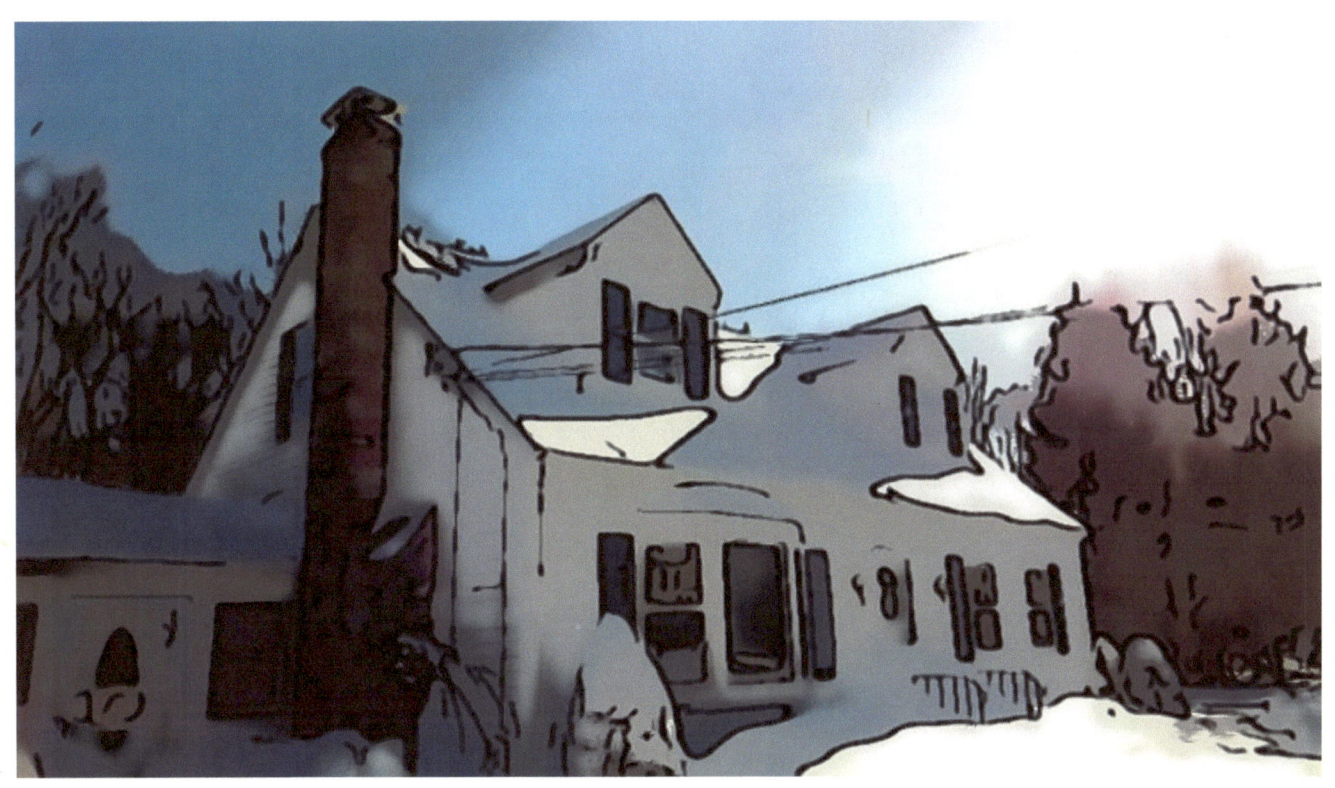

Now I will tell you
   About playing in snow.
As long as we are careful,
   Then we're able to go.

The snow did white shine,
   It was too deep to play.
So we sat in the house,
   All that cold snow filled day.

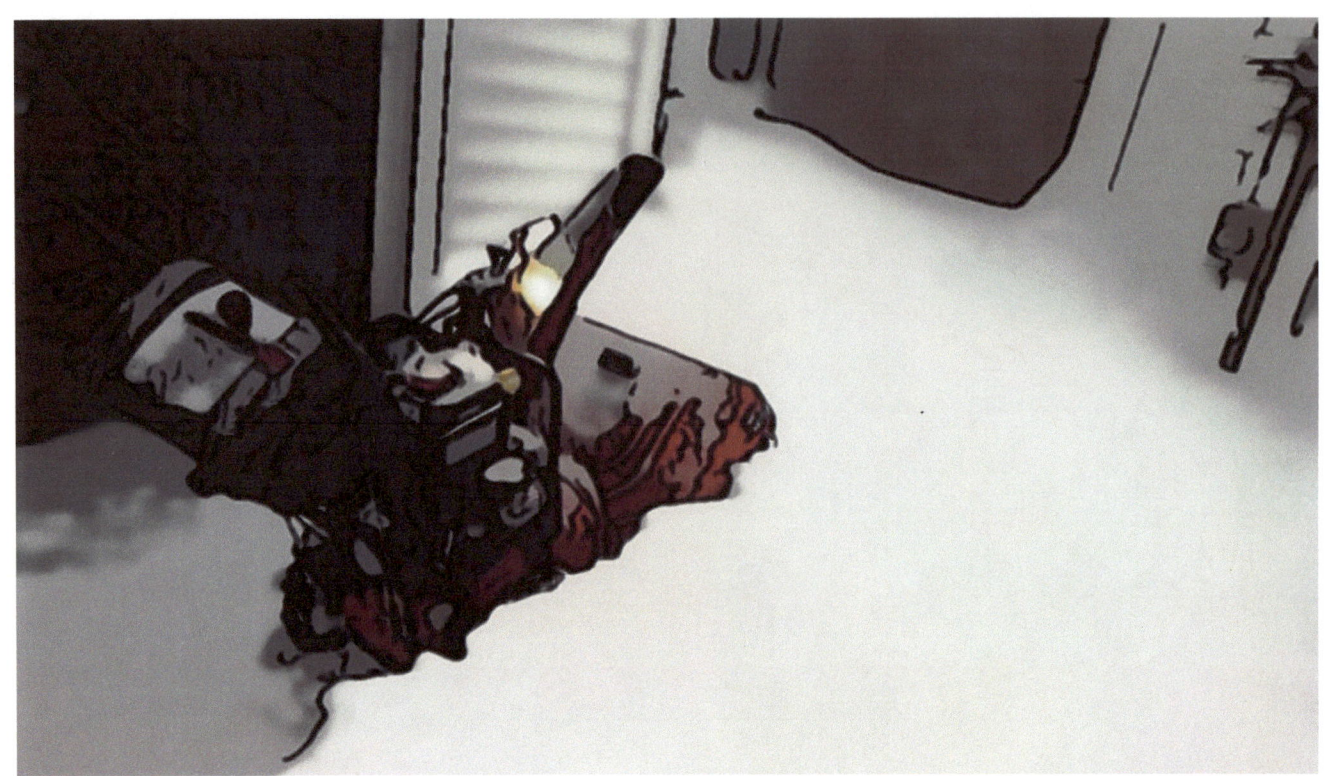

I sat there with Adina,
  I just sat there, alone with her!
And I said "I wish we could
  Use that big snow blower!!"

But all we could do was to
  Sit,
   Sit,
    Sit,
     Sit!
And we did NOT like it,
  Not one little bit!

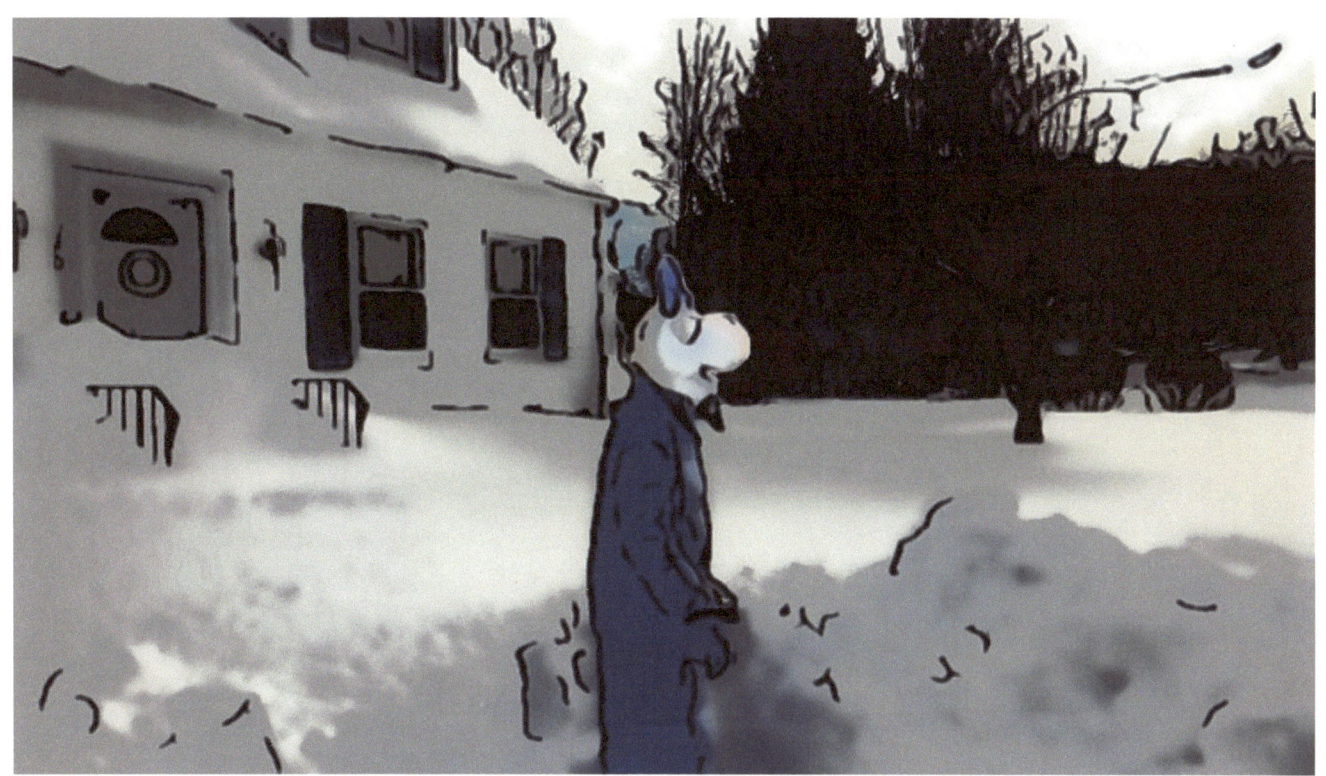

BUMP And then
   Something went bump!
How that bump
   Made us jump!

We looked!   Then we saw him
   Shovel snow and then DUMP!
We looked.   And we saw
   The Moose with the pump

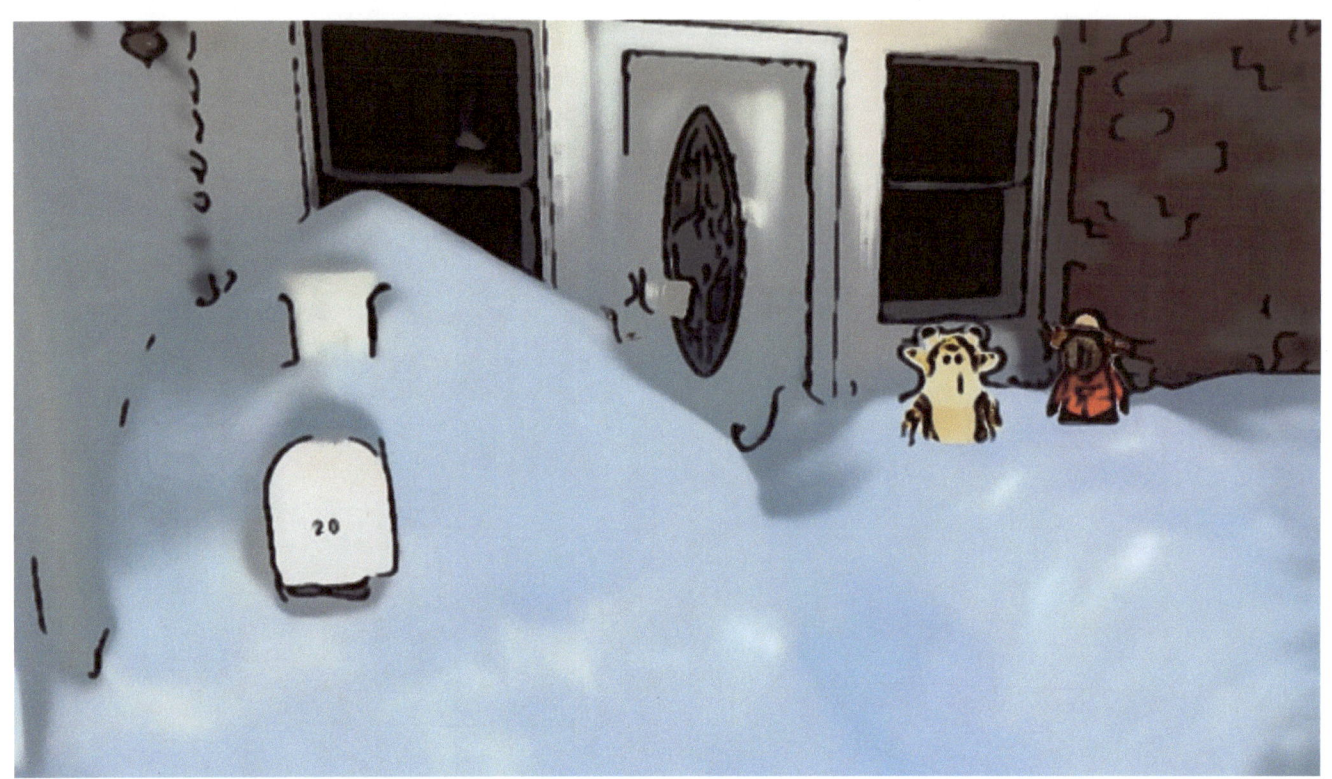

He said to us
  "Why do you look at me sad.
Working in the snow
  Is quite good, so be glad.

Snow is a blessing,
  It is all water you see.
Get on your snowsuits
  And come clean up with me"

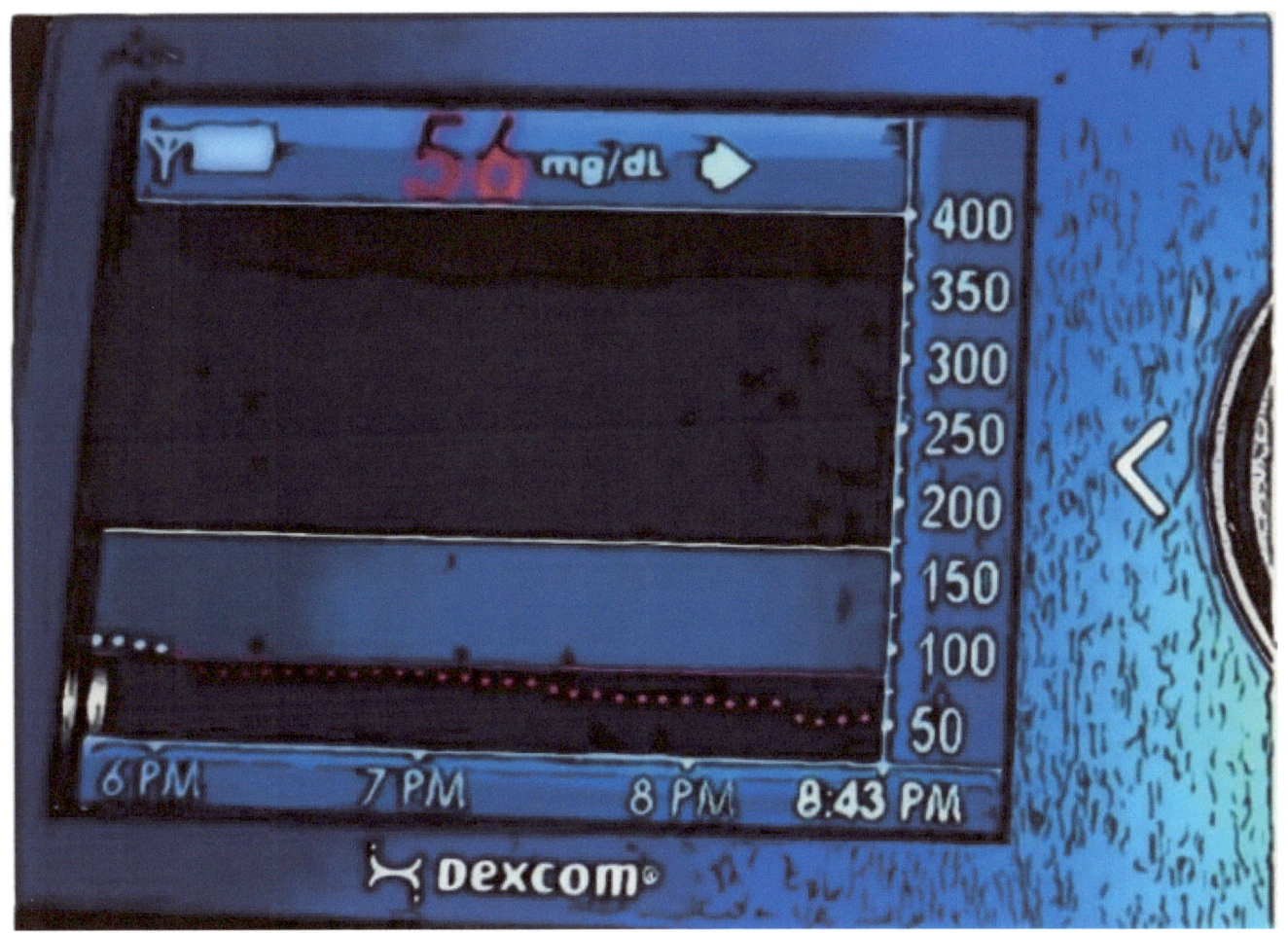

I said, "Our mother said don't
　Go out in the snow
Because my sugar may fall
　And no one will know"

"Your mother is right," he said,
　If no one is around.
But you've got a sensor,
　Which will make a loud sound"

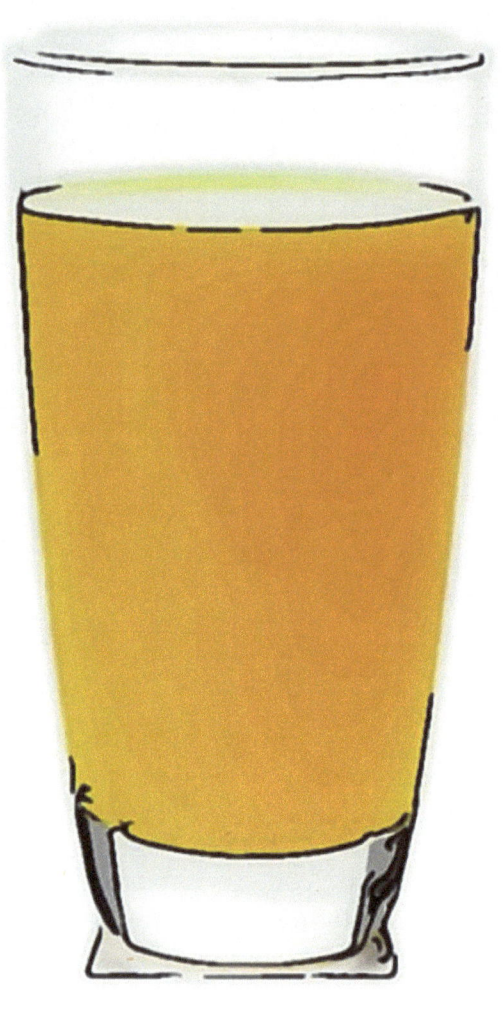
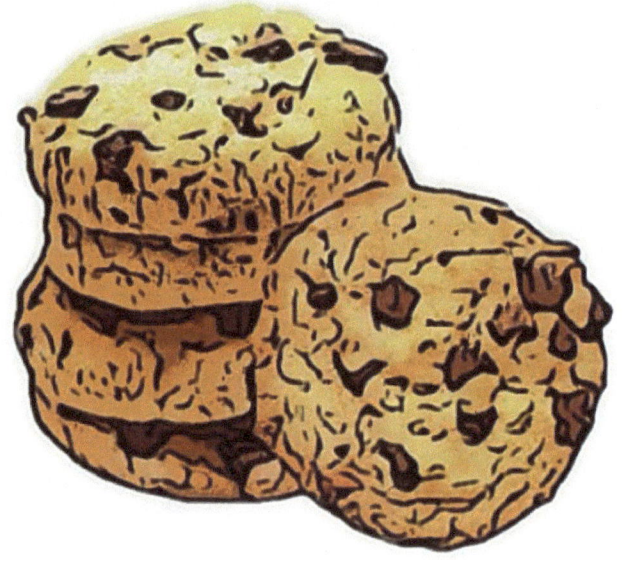

"I'll hear it and so
   Your sister will too
And we'll get you some juice
   Or a small cookie or two"

"You shouldn't be afraid
   To try doing something new.
As long as your sugar is OK
   And your parents let you."

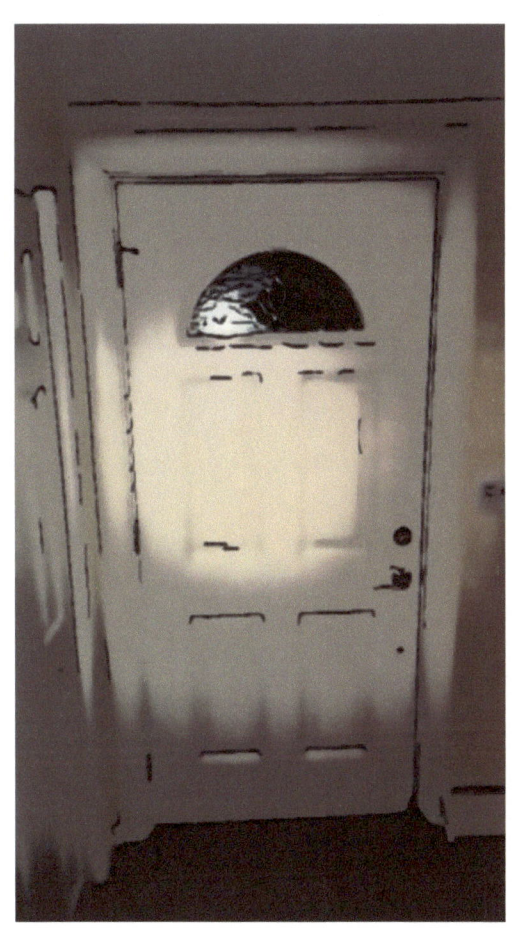

But my sister said "No! No!
 Make that Moose go away!
Tell that Moose with the Pump
 We do NOT want to play!"

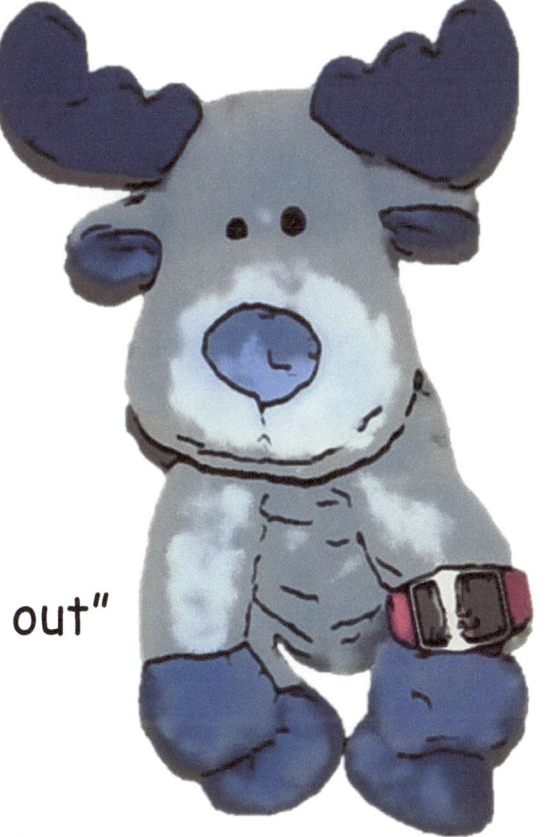

"You should stay in here
 You should not go about
You should stay here inside
 It would be dangerous to go out"

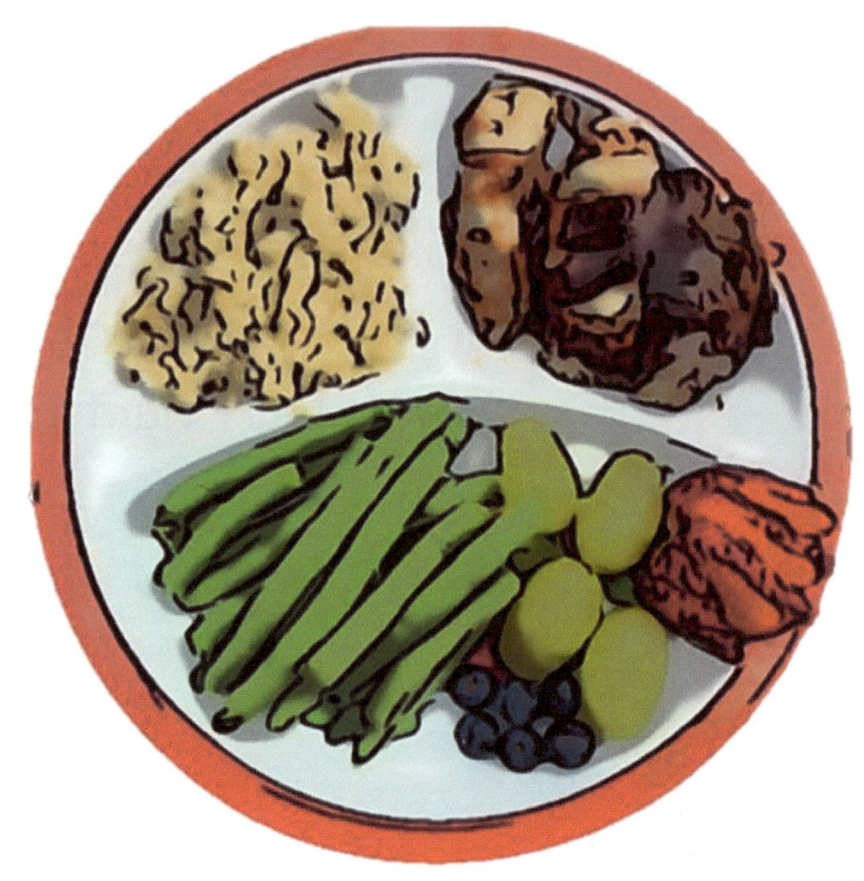

"Now! Now! Have no fear.
   Have no fear! Don't be in a dump.
My ideas are not bad,"
   Said the Moose with the Pump.

"Why, we can have
   Lots of good fun, if you wish,
Your sugar you'll control
   Just count the food in each dish"

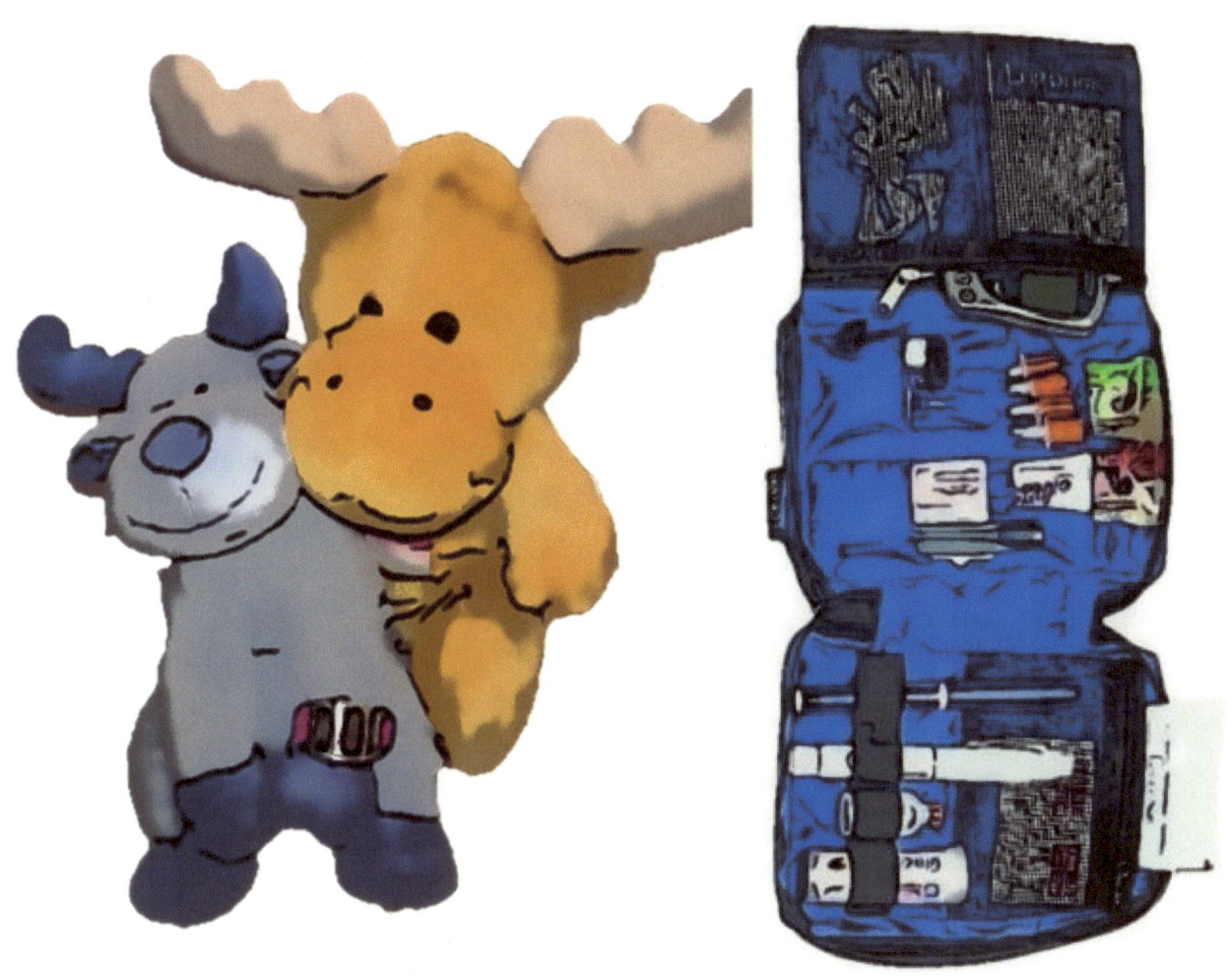

He looked and he said,
   "Ask your mom if you could."
We asked and she said
   "Go with the moose, he is good!"

I've got my kit
   With pump supplies, insulin,
Syringes, glucose meter,
   And cookies within

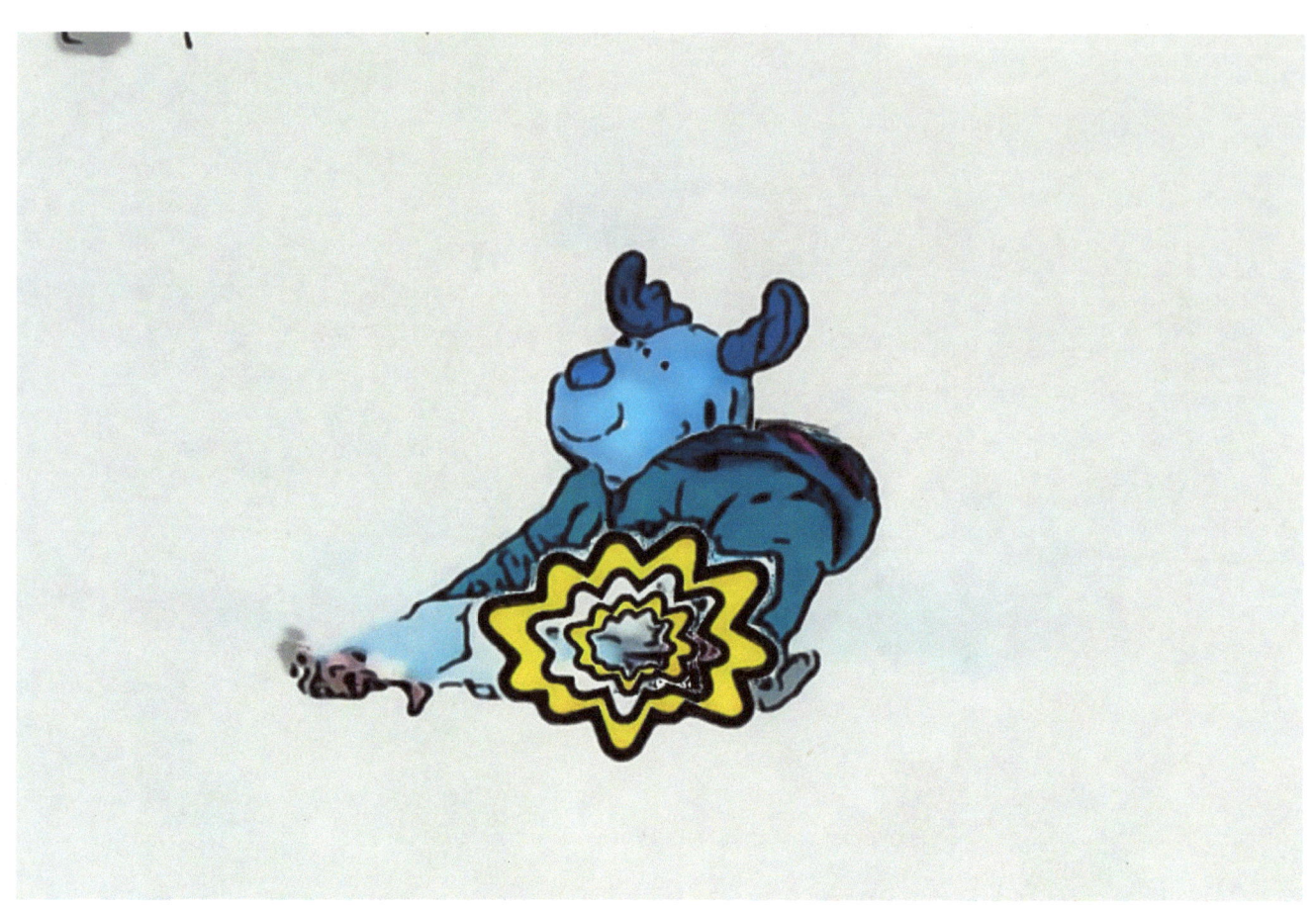

My blood sugar may fall
   When playing in snow.
But my sensor will warn me
   If it falls too low.

So off I went,
   With my friends to play.
To clean the snow
   From sidewalk and driveway.

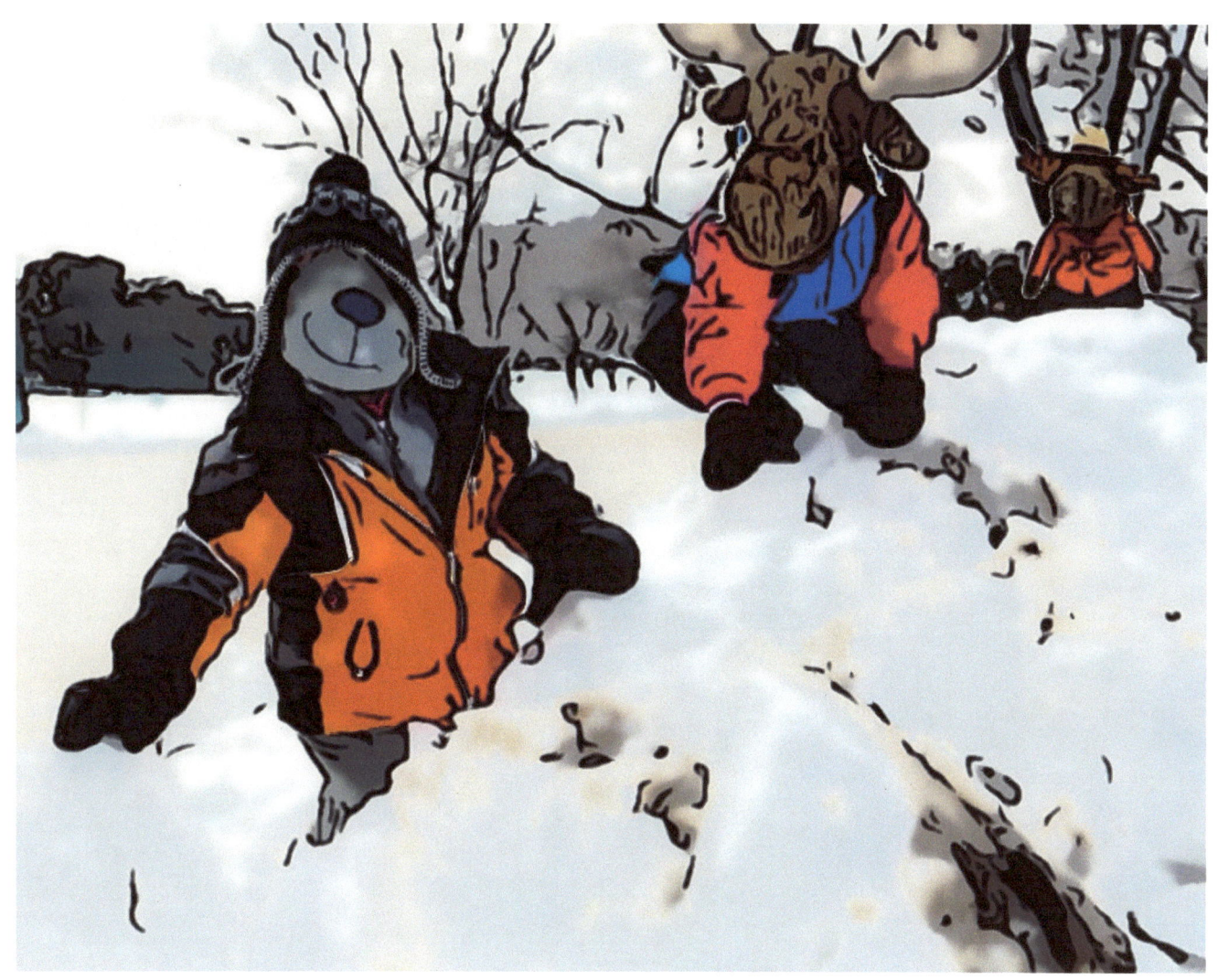

We got on our sweaters
    Jackets, snow pants and socks warm
Snow boots tied tight
    To protect us from the storm

I have to be careful
    When going out in the cold
I must dress in layers
    Just as I've been told

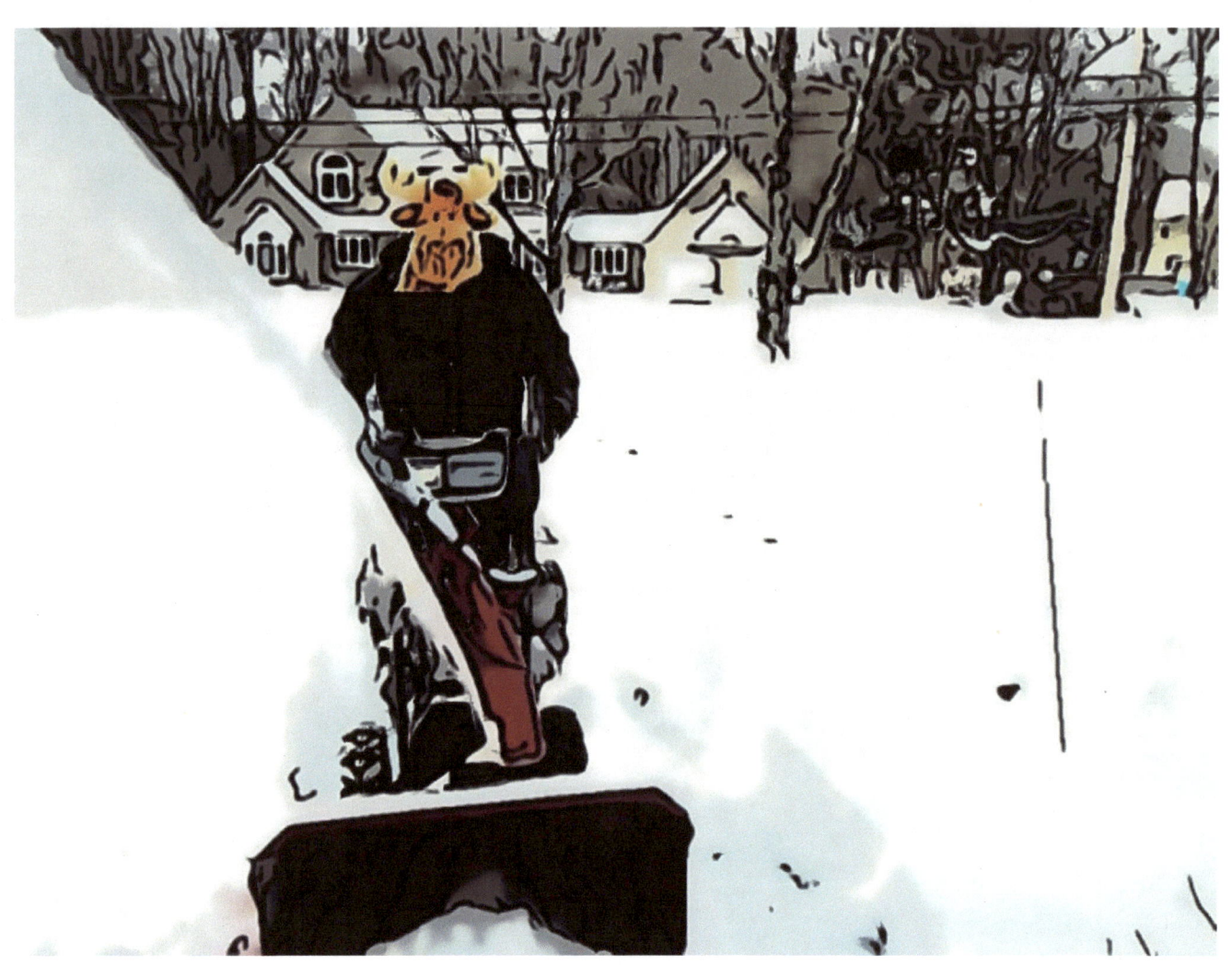

Then the moose took the blower
   And started to blow
He cleared off the driveway
   From all of the snow

He even let me try
   He held my hands tight
So I helped clean the driveway
   From the snow on that night

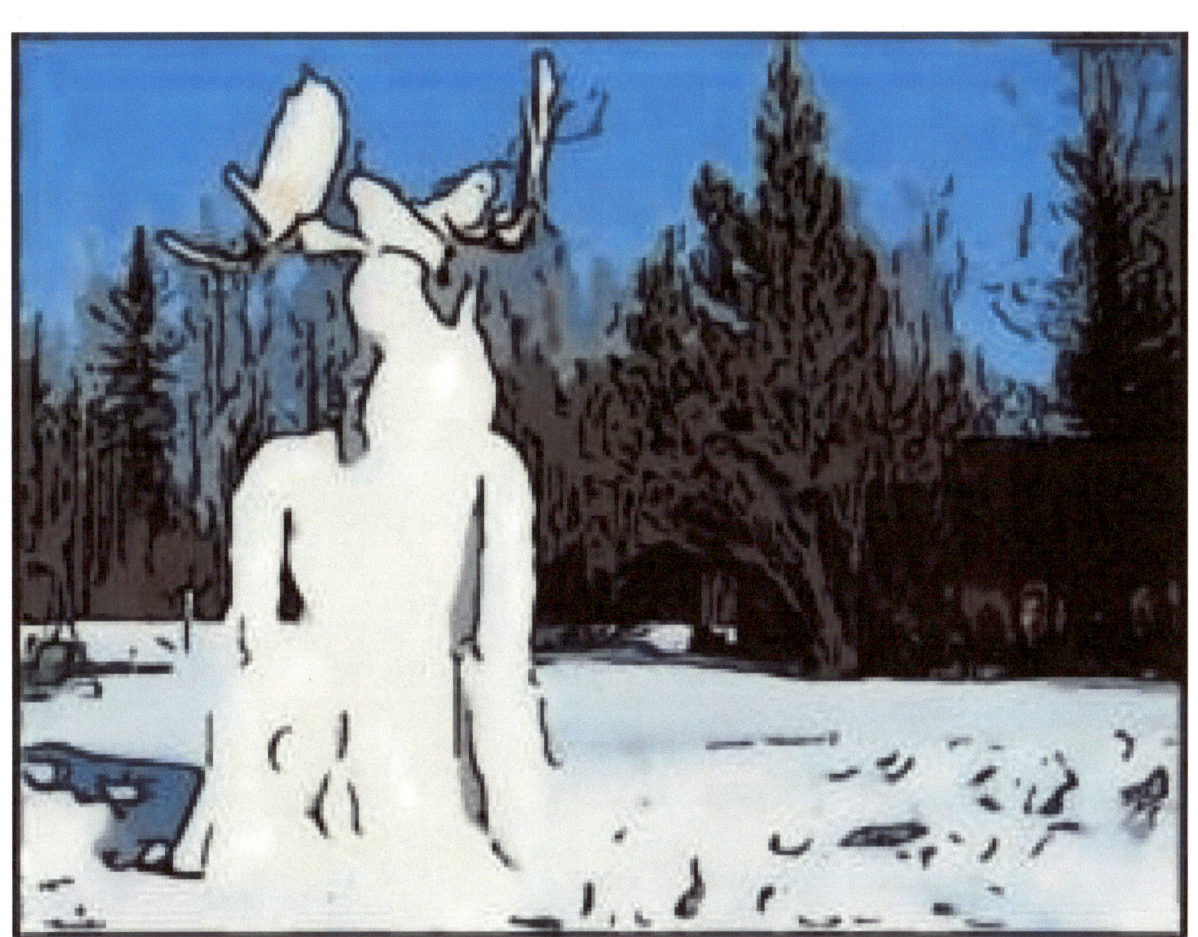

"Let me play myself", I cried out,
 "This is no fun at all.
Let me try making snowballs,
 I'll be careful and not fall.

"Have no fear" said the moose,
 "You shouldn't be scared to fall.
Just have fun in the snow,
 Let's make a snow moose so tall"

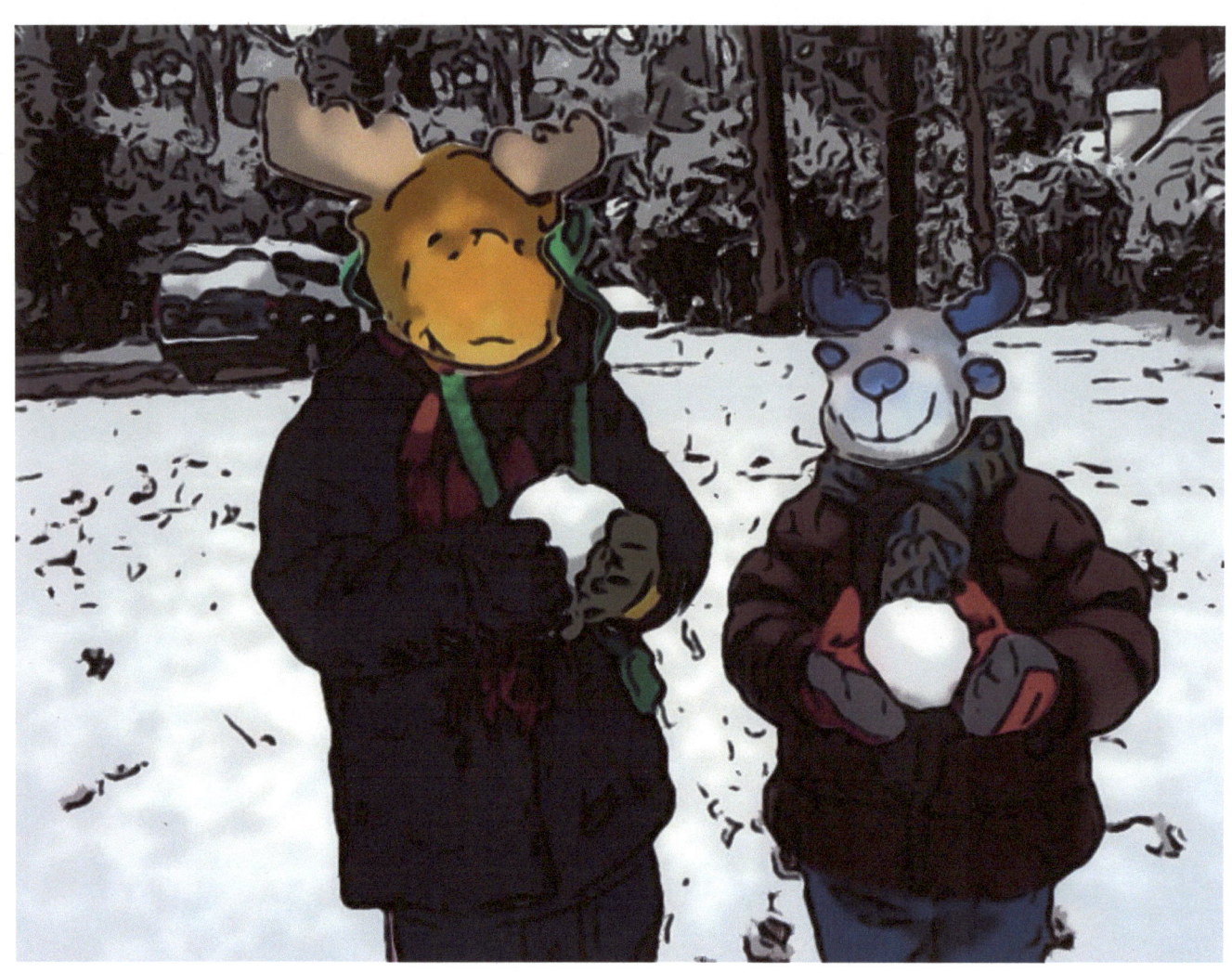

"With the snow in your hands
    You can roll a snow head
Then roll logs for his legs
    And a pump for his meds"

Look at you, look at you
    Look at you Now!
It is fun to have fun
    As long as you know how

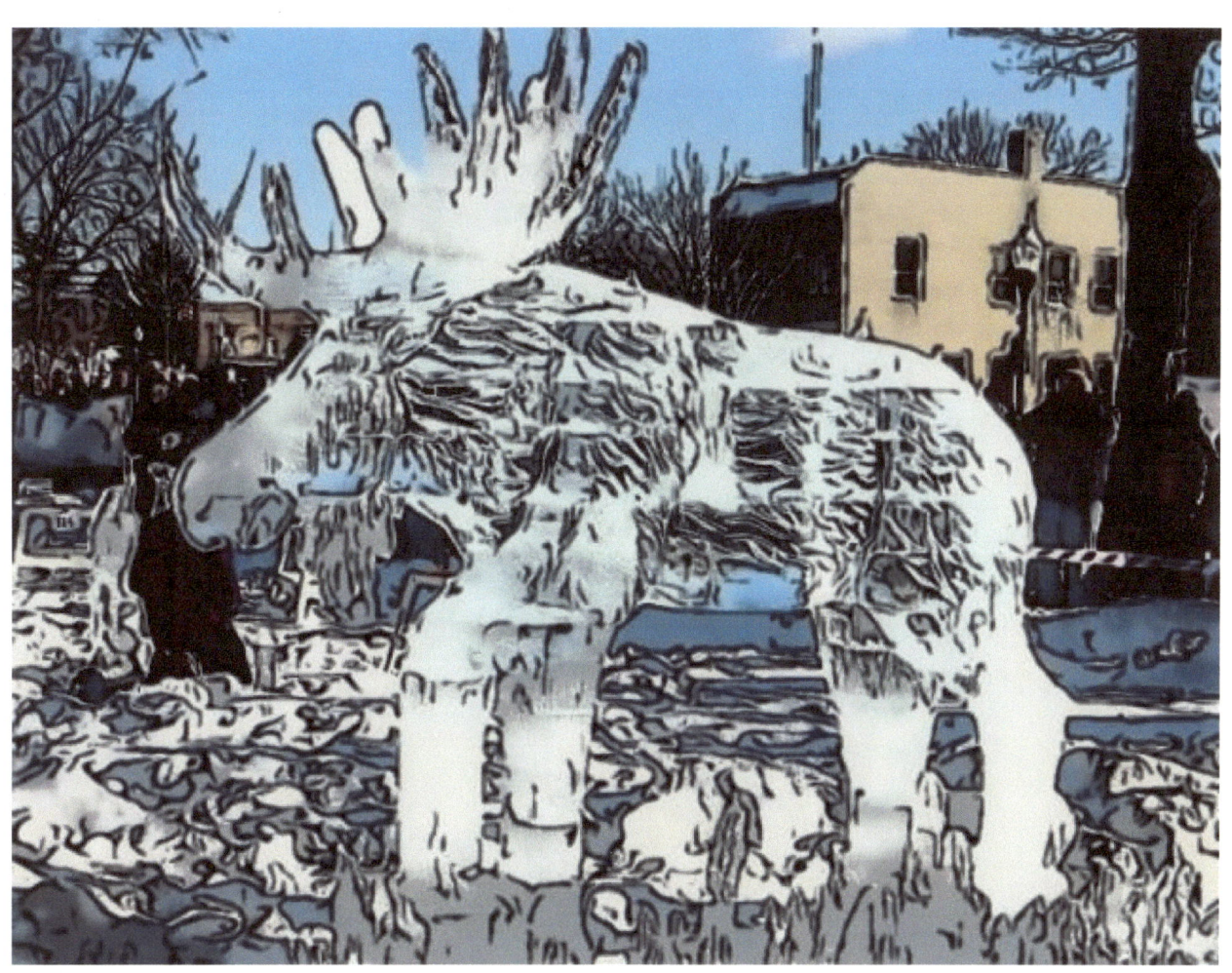

We made a snow head
   And eyes ears and nose
And a huge snow moose body
   And snow feet and toes

So we cleaned up the snow
   And built a big snow moose
With icicle antlers
   And his pump hanging loose

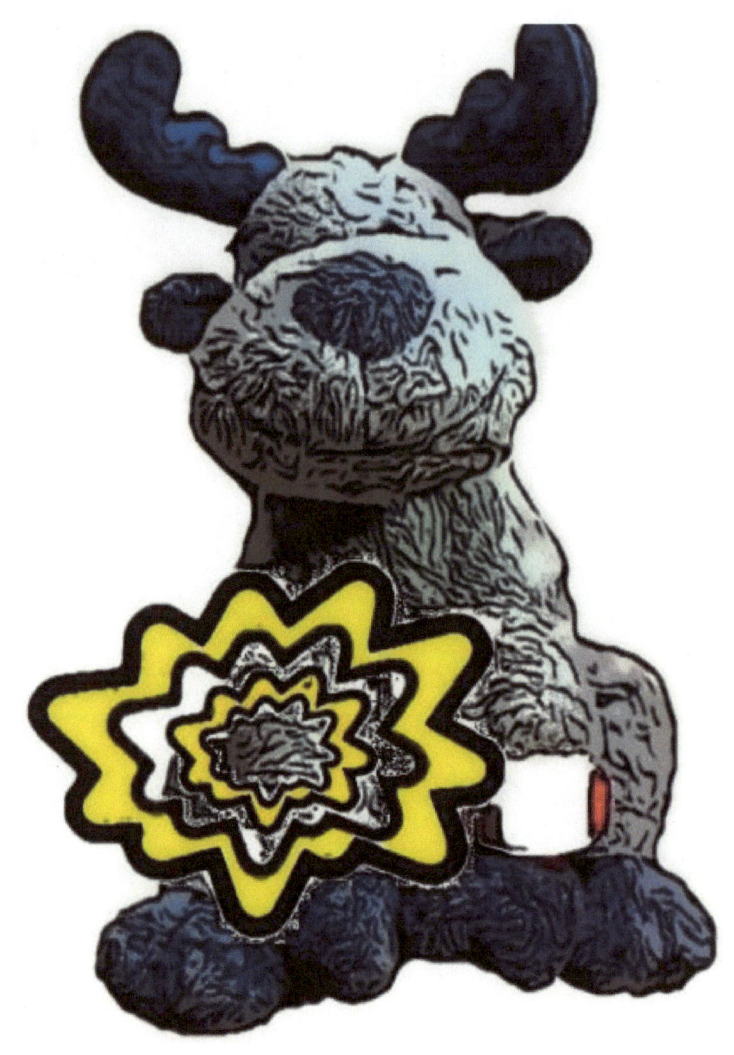

When we were out
   My sensor did ring
My sugar was low
   I must stop everything

I get something to eat
   Then wait 'till I'm OK
Just a few minutes
   And then I can play

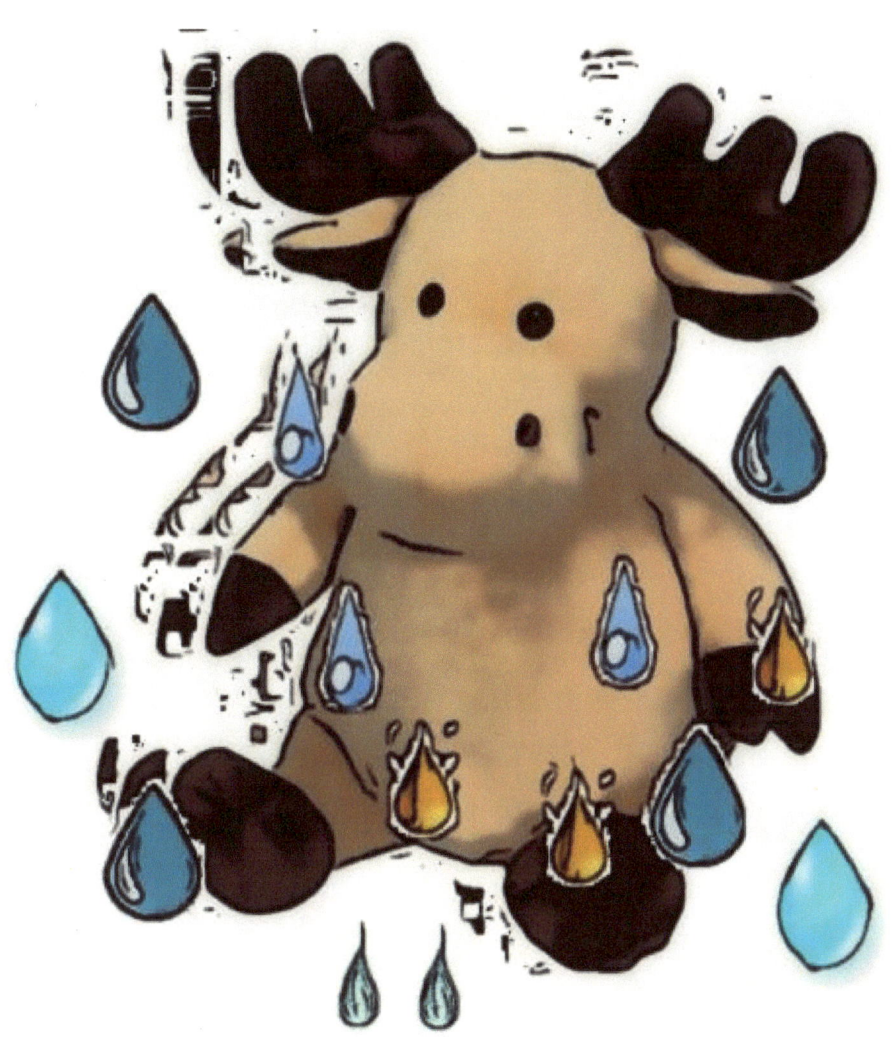

The moose taught me tricks
   Like how I'll feel when I'm low
And when I feel that I am
   Quickly get food, don't be slow

If I'm shaky or cold
   Or find it hard to speak
Or wild and crazy
   Or tired and weak

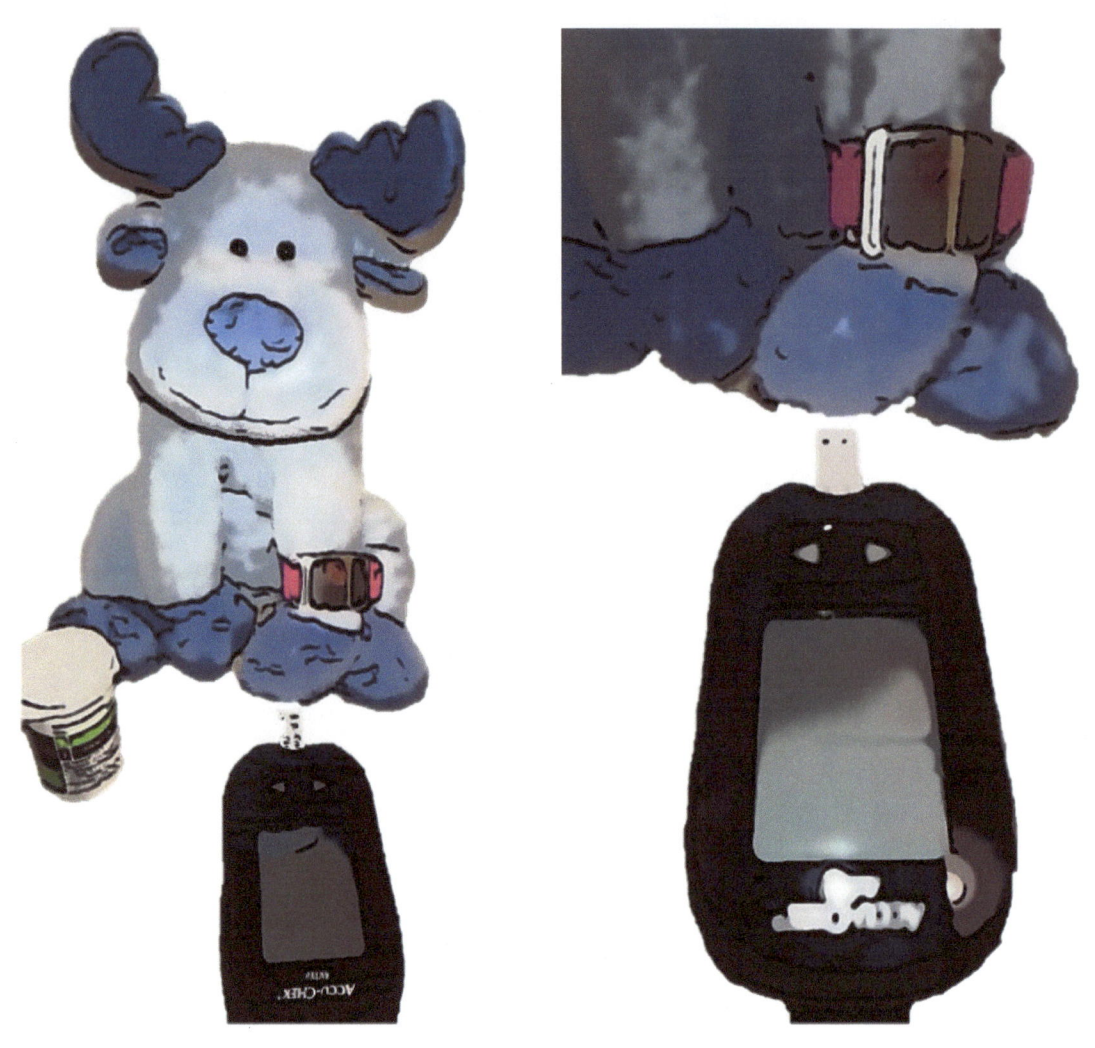

When things don't seem normal
   It's always best to just see
If my blood sugar is off
   And to take care of me

The moose helped me out
   On that cold snowy day
he then began teaching
   And for a while did stay

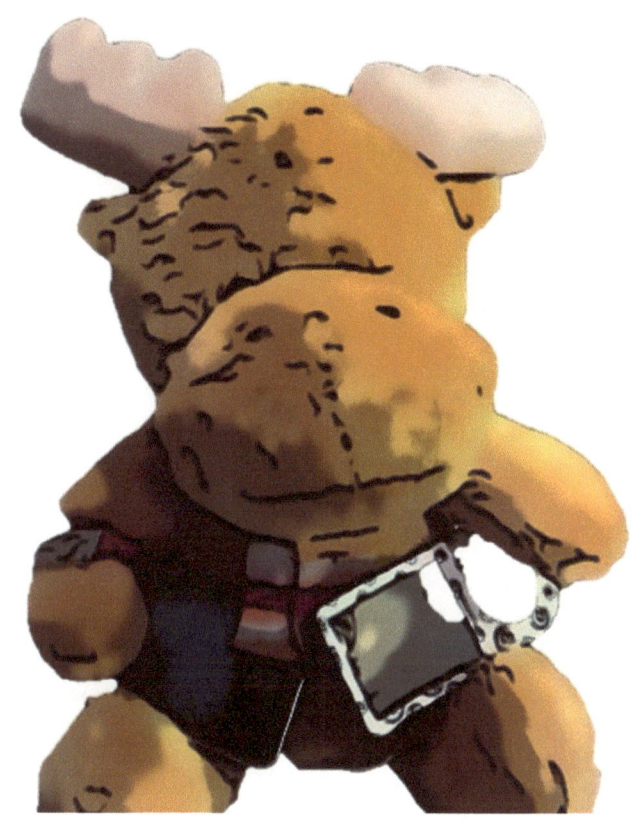

You must always have
   Your sensor with you
And your pump must be full
   And both charged up too

Filling your pump
   With insulin for you
Isn't that hard
   When you're old enough to

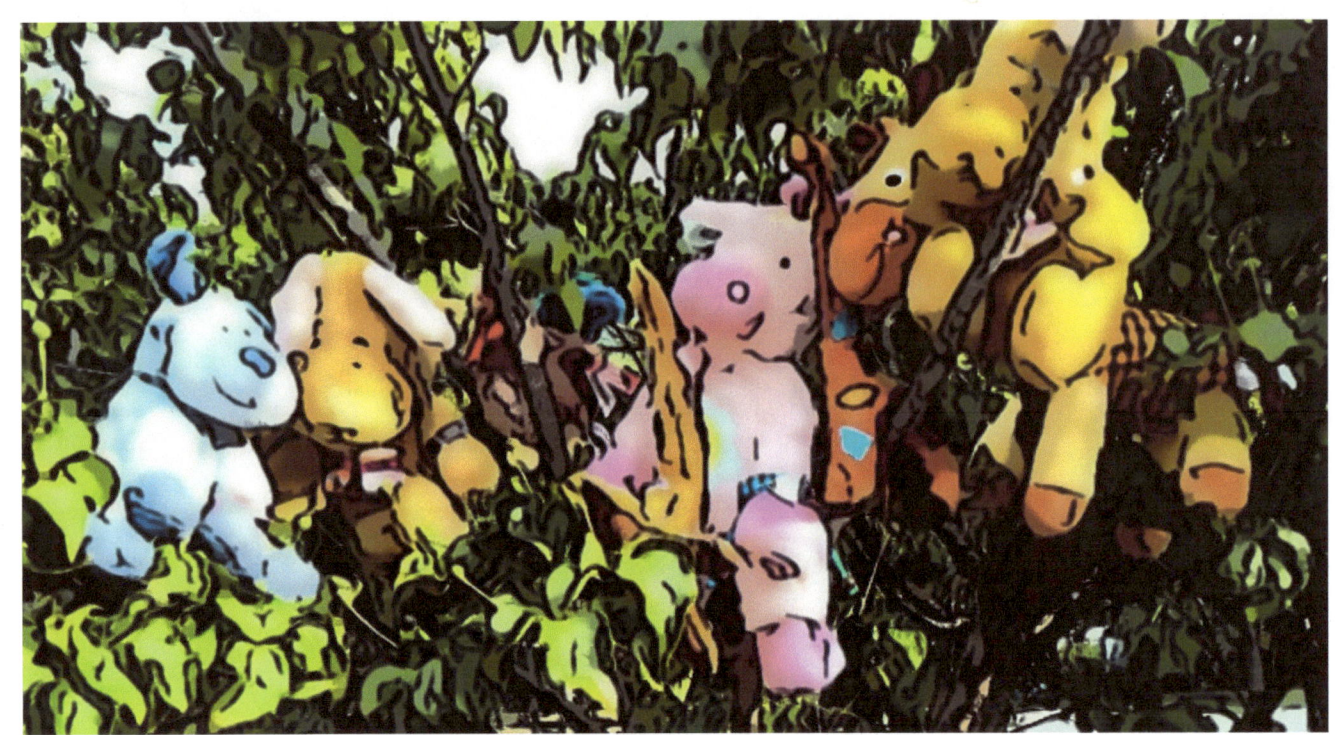

Your mom or your dad
  Can show you the way,
To put in a new set
  So it will stay.

When playing be careful
  When moving about,
That the pump is secure
  And doesn't fall out.

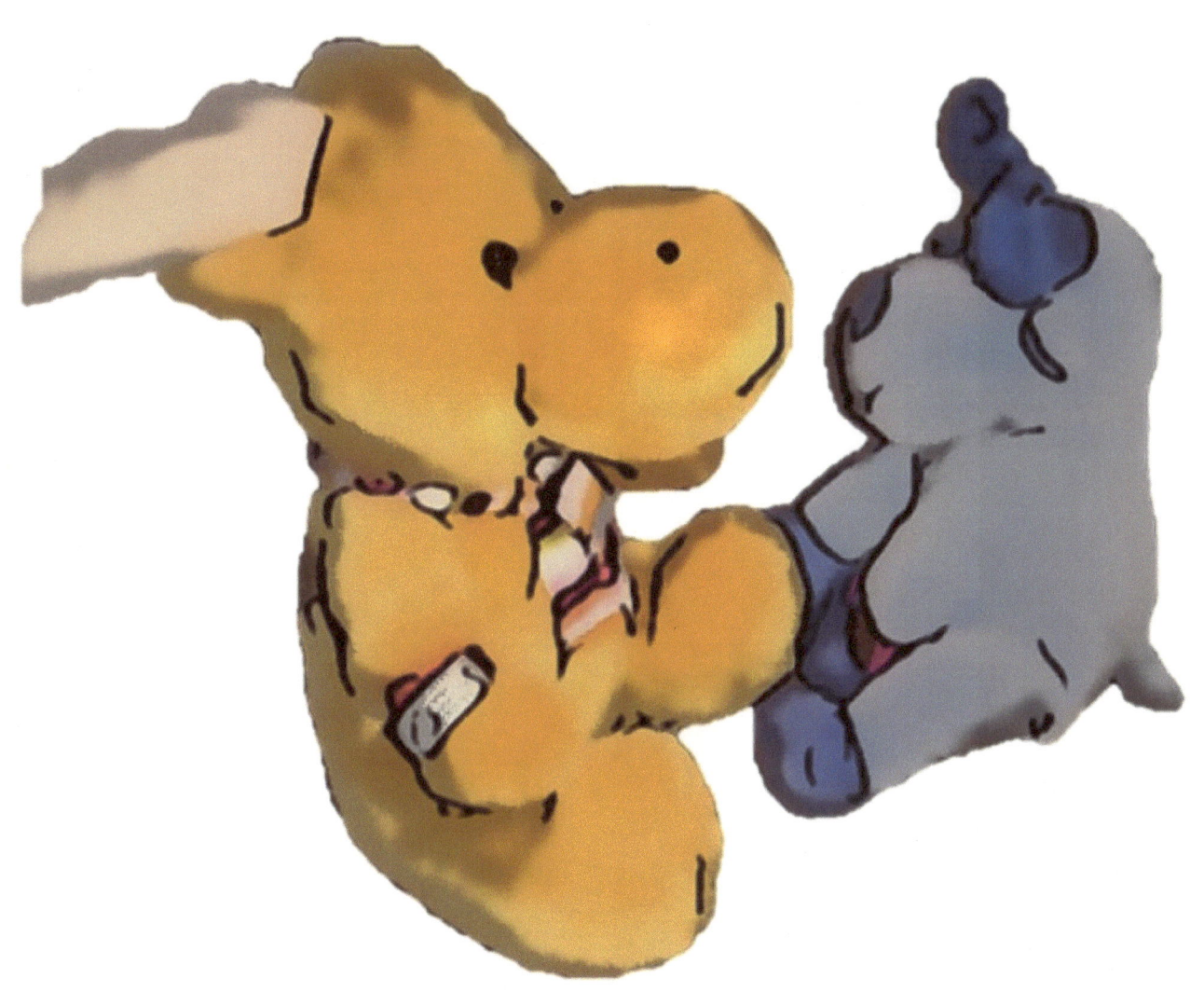

And now you can play
   Out in the snow
You know what to do
   To prepare to go

We'll continue to learn
   About school, spring and the gym
And after school's over
   This summer we'll swim

The Moose with the Pump: A book for children with type 1 diabetes

Learning to Live with Diabetes for Children Book Series (3 Books)

Endorsements:

"*The moose with the pump*" is an endearing story which shows children with diabetes they do not have to be afraid to play in the snow with their friends.

The book illustrates the story using pictures of stuffed animals "utilizing" insulin pumps, glucose sensors and other machines associated with diabetes care and demonstrates a real-life situation that guides children to take care of themselves.

This book is a good follow up to the original "*I can help take care of Me*" and would be a great story to read a young child diagnosed with diabetes.

Sara Chana Hecht, RN Case Manager and Wellness Programs

I had the privilege of reading this book with an objective eye from living with Diabetes successfully after 55 years and also as a retired BSN, CDE. I only wish I had this book to help Children and their parents years ago. Knowledge bans the fear, and releases enthusiasm for life.

Brenda Trexler McGowan, retired BSN. CDE.

The Moose with the Pump by Yerachmiel Altman is about David Jacob, the little blue moose who has type 1 diabetes. His parents tell him that he need not be scared as they will not let him down and, with the right information, he will be safe and sound. They tell him that they will help him to learn to keep his sugar good all day using shots, blood tests, pumps, and sensors. His big sister, Adina, also knows how to take care of him. Winter is coming and David wants to play in the snow and be safe at the same time. Will David be able to play in the snow? What happens when they meet The Moose with the Pump? Read the story to find out!

The story is adorable and shows how children with type 1 diabetes can play safely in the snow. It is informative to many parents and it also guides children to take care of themselves by showing them how to use insulin pumps, glucose sensors, and other machines associated with diabetes care. The story is written in a poetic manner, making it lyrical and giving the story a good pace and movement. The illustrations are colorful and endearing and they bring the characters and scenes alive. It is a good bedtime storybook and also good for read aloud sessions in classrooms and school libraries as it gives information about how to take care when one has type 1 diabetes.

Reviewed By Mamta Madhavan for Readers' Favorite

CPSIA information can be obtained
at www.ICGtesting.com
Printed in the USA
LVHW072346191119
637879LV00009B/296/P